TABLE OF CONTENTS

INTRODUCTION

CHAPTER ONE

CHAPTER TWO

CHAPTER THREE

CHAPTER FOUR

INTRODUCTION

In recent years, vaping has transitioned from a niche trend to a global phenomenon, drawing millions of individuals with its promise of a cleaner, more customizable alternative to smoking. Unlike traditional cigarettes, which are often associated with health risks and environmental concerns, vaping introduces a modern approach to nicotine consumption, blending sleek technology with a vast array of flavor options. This new method of inhaling nicotine has not only changed the way people approach smoking cessation but also reshaped recreational nicotine use, offering a level of personalization that traditional cigarettes cannot match.

As curiosity about vaping continues to rise, so does the complexity of the devices and the variety of products available. From advanced mod setups that cater to enthusiasts to simple pod systems designed for beginners, vaping presents a diverse range of experiences tailored to individual preferences. This evolution in nicotine consumption brings with it both opportunities and challenges, making it crucial to understand the nuances of how to vape effectively and responsibly.

Whether you are considering vaping as a potential alternative to smoking, exploring its myriad flavors, or simply curious about this technological shift, this guide aims to provide a comprehensive overview of the vaping world. We will delve into the different types of devices, the science behind vaping, and practical tips for getting started, ensuring that you can navigate this exciting landscape with confidence and knowledge.

CHAPTER ONE

E-CIGARETTES

An electronic cigarette, commonly known as an e-cigarette or vape, is a sophisticated device designed to replicate the experience of smoking traditional tobacco. This device is composed of several key components: an atomizer, a power source typically in the form of a battery, and a container such as a cartridge or tank that holds the e-liquid. Unlike conventional cigarettes, which produce smoke through the combustion of tobacco, e-cigarettes generate vapor, hence the term "vaping" is used to describe their usage.

The core component, the atomizer, serves as a heating element that vaporizes the e-liquid contained within the device. This liquid solution, often referred to as e-liquid, is transformed into an aerosol consisting of tiny droplets that are then inhaled by the user. The primary constituents of this vapor are propylene glycol and/or glycerin, which may be combined with nicotine and various flavorings to enhance the user's experience. The precise composition of the vapor can vary significantly, influenced by factors such as the specific formulation of the e-liquid and the individual usage patterns of the consumer. This variability underscores the complexity of e-cigarette technology and its capacity to deliver a customizable alternative to traditional smoking methods.

E-cigarettes, also known as vapes, are designed to be activated either by taking a puff or by pressing a button. This functionality makes their use intuitive and convenient. Certain models are crafted to resemble traditional cigarettes, while the majority of e-cigarettes are designed to be reusable, offering a more sustainable option for users.

Nicotine, the primary addictive component in e-cigarettes, has a high potential for addiction, leading users to develop both physical and psychological dependencies. Despite extensive research, the long-term health implications of e-cigarette use remain unclear. This uncertainty is partly due to the challenge of isolating the effects of vaping from those of smoking, as many individuals engage in both behaviors. The relatively recent advent of e-cigarettes means that they have not been in widespread use long enough to allow for definitive long-term studies.

While vaping is generally considered to be significantly less harmful than smoking traditional cigarettes, it is not without risks. The vapor produced by e-cigarettes contains fewer toxins and at lower concentrations compared to cigarette smoke. However, it also includes certain harmful substances that are not present in traditional cigarette smoke.

E-cigarettes have been shown to be more effective than traditional nicotine replacement therapy (NRT) products in aiding smoking cessation. Nevertheless, e-cigarettes have not undergone the same rigorous testing as most NRT products. Consequently, there are concerns about their safety and efficacy. Health warnings associated with e-cigarettes might also encourage smokers to reconsider and potentially cease vaping. This highlights the need for continued research and regulatory scrutiny to ensure the safety and effectiveness of e-cigarettes as smoking cessation aids.

HISTORY

The assertion that the modern e-cigarette was invented in 2003 by Chinese pharmacist Hon Lik is widely accepted, but the concept of nicotine aerosol generation predates this by several decades. Tobacco companies had been exploring similar technologies since at least 1963.

Early Innovations and Challenges: 1920s–1990s

The origins of electronic vaporization can be traced back to 1927 when Joseph Robinson filed a patent application for an electronic vaporizer intended for medicinal use. Although Robinson's patent was approved in 1930, the device was never brought to market. This early patent described a method for holding medicinal compounds that could be electrically or otherwise heated to produce vapors for inhalation. Subsequent patents in 1934 and 1936 also explored similar technologies.

One of the earliest e-cigarette concepts can be attributed to American inventor Herbert A. Gilbert. In 1963, Gilbert filed a patent application for a "smokeless non-tobacco cigarette" designed to replace the burning of tobacco and paper with heated, moist, flavored air. This invention produced flavored steam but did not include nicotine. Gilbert's patent was granted in 1965, but his device did not gain traction or commercialization at the time, partly due to the prevailing popularity of traditional smoking. In 2013, Gilbert noted that modern electric cigarettes closely follow the basic design principles outlined in his original patent.

Another significant development in the evolution of non-combustible nicotine products occurred in 1986 with the introduction of the Favor cigarette by Advanced Tobacco Products, a public company. Conceptualized by Phil Ray, one of the founders of Datapoint Corporation and a pioneer in microprocessor technology, Favor was a plastic, smoke-free product designed to resemble a conventional cigarette. It contained a filter paper saturated with liquid nicotine, allowing users to inhale a small dose without combustion or smoke. Despite its innovative design, Favor did not achieve commercial success.

The Favor cigarettes were marketed in California and several states in the Southwestern United States as a solution for smokers seeking alternatives in areas where smoking was either restricted or prohibited. The promotional strategy emphasized that the product was specifically designed for smokers who faced limitations on where they could smoke.

In 1987, the U.S. Food and Drug Administration (FDA) asserted its regulatory authority over products similar to e-cigarettes, which led to significant implications for the Favor cigarettes. Advanced Tobacco Products, the company behind Favor, did not contest the FDA's Warning Letter and subsequently discontinued the product's distribution.

Interestingly, the term "vaping," now commonly associated with electronic cigarettes, was coined by Brenda Coffee, the wife of Phil Ray, one of the inventors of the Favor cigarette.

In a later development, Philip Morris launched the MarkTen e-cigarette through its division, NuMark, in 2013. This product was the result of Philip Morris's extensive research and development efforts on e-cigarette technology, which had been ongoing since 1990.

Modern electronic cigarettes, as we know them today, can be traced back to the work of Hon Lik, a Chinese pharmacist and inventor who was previously employed as a research pharmacist for a company specializing in ginseng products. Despite earlier attempts at developing nicotine delivery systems, Hon Lik is widely recognized for his contributions to the modern e-cigarette.

Motivated by a personal tragedy, the death of his father, a heavy smoker who succumbed to lung cancer, Hon Lik sought to create a safer alternative to traditional smoking. In 2001, he conceived the idea of using a high-frequency piezoelectric ultrasound-emitting element to vaporize a pressurized jet of liquid nicotine, thereby producing a vapor that mimics the experience of smoke. However, Hon discovered that resistance heating provided superior results and faced the challenge of miniaturizing the device to a practical size.

Hon Lik envisioned the e-cigarette as a revolutionary alternative to smoking, likening its impact to that of the digital camera supplanting the analogue camera. Despite his innovative achievement, Hon Lik himself did not fully quit smoking and currently uses both traditional cigarettes and e-cigarettes.

Hon Lik, credited with developing the modern e-cigarette, registered a patent for his design in 2003. He is widely recognized for creating the first commercially successful electronic cigarette. This innovation was first introduced to the Chinese domestic market in 2004, and shortly thereafter, versions of the e-cigarette began appearing in the US market, primarily sold online by smaller marketing firms. The e-cigarette made its European debut in 2006, followed by its US introduction in 2007. In November 2007, Hon's employer, Golden Dragon Holdings, registered an international patent for the design. Later that month, the company rebranded as Ruyan, meaning "like smoke" in Chinese, and commenced exporting its products.

Despite the innovation, many US and Chinese e-cigarette manufacturers replicated Hon's design without authorization, resulting in limited financial compensation for his invention, although some US companies have settled out of court. Ruyan later changed its name to Dragonite International Limited. By 2014, most e-cigarettes had transitioned to battery-powered heating elements, moving away from the original ultrasonic technology.

Initially, early e-cigarettes did not fully meet user expectations. However, the technology continued to evolve beyond the first-generation three-part device. In 2007, British entrepreneurs Umer and Tariq Sheikh introduced the cartomizer, a mechanism integrating the heating coil into the liquid chamber. This innovation was launched in the UK in 2008 under the Gamucci brand and has since been widely adopted by "cigalike" brands. Concurrently, enthusiasts began modifying devices to improve performance and aesthetics, giving rise to the hobby known as "modding." The first notable mod, known as the "screwdriver," was developed by Ted and Matt Rogers in 2008, featuring a larger battery and improved functionality.

The screwdriver's success generated substantial interest and demand for customizable e-cigarettes. This led manufacturers to produce devices with interchangeable components. In 2009, Joyetech introduced the eGo series, which offered similar power to the screwdriver model along with a user-activated switch. Additionally, the clearomizer was invented in 2009, evolving from the cartomizer design to include the wicking material, e-liquid chamber, and atomizer coil within a single transparent component. The clearomizer allowed users to monitor the liquid level and was soon followed by the introduction of replaceable atomizer coils and variable voltage batteries. By early

2012, clearomizers and eGo batteries had become popular and best-selling customizable e-cigarette components.

Initially, international tobacco companies regarded e-cigarettes as a mere trend. However, recognizing the potential for e-cigarettes to establish a new market sector and possibly make traditional tobacco products obsolete, these companies began investing heavily in this emerging field. They started to produce their own e-cigarette brands and acquire existing e-cigarette firms. Notably, major tobacco corporations purchased some of the largest e-cigarette companies available. For instance, Lorillard Inc. acquired blu eCigs, a leading US e-cigarette manufacturer, for $135 million in April 2012.

British American Tobacco (BAT) was the first tobacco company to enter the UK e-cigarette market. In July 2013, BAT launched its e-cigarette brand, Vype. Similarly, Imperial

Tobacco's Fontem Ventures purchased the intellectual property from Hon Lik through Dragonite International Limited for $75 million in 2013 and introduced the Puritane e-cigarette in partnership with Boots UK. On October 1, 2013, Lorillard Inc. continued its acquisition spree by purchasing the UK-based e-cigarette company SKYCIG. Following this acquisition, SKYCIG was rebranded as blu, consolidating Lorillard's presence in the e-cigarette market.

On February 3, 2014, Altria Group, Inc., one of the major players in the tobacco industry, acquired the well-known e-cigarette brand Green Smoke for $110 million. This acquisition was completed in April 2014 and included an additional $20 million in incentive payments. In addition to acquiring Green Smoke, Altria markets its own e-cigarette brand, MarkTen. Meanwhile, Reynolds American has entered the e-cigarette market with its Vuse product.

Philip Morris, the world's largest tobacco company, expanded its e-cigarette portfolio by purchasing the UK's Nicocigs in June 2014. Additionally, Japan Tobacco acquired the US-based Logic e-cigarette brand on April 30, 2015, and also purchased the UK E-Lites brand in June 2014. Furthermore, on July 15, 2014, Lorillard sold its blu brand to Imperial Tobacco in a substantial deal valued at $7.1 billion.

As of 2018, the vast majority of e-cigarettes, approximately 95%, were manufactured in China. In the United Kingdom, where the predominant method of vaping involves refillable devices and e-liquids, there has been notable support from the National Health Service (NHS) and various other medical organizations. These bodies now recognize e-cigarettes as a potentially effective smoking cessation tool. Consequently, the number of individuals using e-cigarettes has reached a record high, with over 3.6 million vapers reported as of June 2021.

19

CHAPTER TWO

CONSTRUCTION

An electronic cigarette, commonly known as an e-cigarette or vape, comprises three primary components: an atomizer, which serves as the heating element; a power source, typically a rechargeable battery; and a container, such as a cartridge or tank, that holds the e-liquid.

The design and functionality of e-cigarettes have undergone significant evolution, leading to the development of various generations of devices. First-generation e-cigarettes, often referred to as "cigalikes," closely mimic the appearance of traditional cigarettes. These early models are typically small and straightforward in design, aiming to provide a familiar experience for smokers transitioning to vaping.

Second-generation e-cigarettes introduced larger devices that diverged from the traditional cigarette aesthetic. These devices offered improved battery life and more substantial vapor production, enhancing the overall vaping experience.

Third-generation devices further advanced the technology, featuring mechanical mods and variable voltage devices. These innovations allowed users to customize their vaping experience by adjusting the power output, resulting in a more personalized and satisfying use.

The fourth-generation of e-cigarettes includes sub-ohm tanks and temperature control features. Sub-ohm tanks, characterized by their electrical resistance of less than one ohm, produce larger vapor clouds and deliver more intense flavors. Temperature control technology ensures a consistent and controlled vaping experience by regulating the coil temperature, preventing dry hits and extending coil life.

In addition to these advancements, there are also pod mod devices that use protonated nicotine, which differs from the free-base nicotine found in earlier generations. Protonated nicotine allows for higher nicotine yields, providing a more potent nicotine delivery while maintaining a smooth throat hit. These pod mod systems are compact and user-friendly, appealing to both new and experienced vapers.

Overall, the evolution of e-cigarette technology reflects ongoing efforts to improve performance, user experience, and satisfaction. Each generation has introduced new features and enhancements, catering to the diverse preferences and needs of the vaping community.

The liquid used in vapor products such as e-cigarettes is referred to as e-liquid or vape juice. E-liquid formulations can vary significantly, but a typical composition consists of 95% propylene glycol and glycerin, with the remaining 5% made up of flavorings, nicotine, and other additives. The flavorings used in e-liquids can be natural, artificial, or organic, catering to a wide range of consumer preferences.

Despite the appeal of various flavors, it's important to note that e-liquids can contain trace amounts of over 80 harmful chemicals, including formaldehyde and metallic nanoparticles. These substances, even in small quantities, raise concerns about the potential health risks associated with e-cigarette use.

The market for e-liquids is extensive, with numerous manufacturers producing a vast array of products. It is estimated that there are more than 15,000 different e-liquid flavors available, reflecting the industry's rapid growth and the diverse tastes of consumers.

Given the potential health risks and the wide variety of products, many countries have implemented regulations to control the contents of e-liquids. In the United States, the Food and Drug Administration (FDA) enforces mandatory manufacturing standards to ensure safety and quality. Additionally, the American E-liquid Manufacturing Standards Association (AEMSA) provides recommended manufacturing standards to guide producers.

In the European Union, e-liquid standards are outlined in the EU Tobacco Products Directive, which sets stringent requirements for product safety and labeling. These regulations aim to protect consumers by ensuring that e-liquids meet specific safety criteria and are produced under controlled conditions.

Overall, the regulation of e-liquids is crucial for maintaining consumer safety and product integrity. As the e-cigarette market continues to evolve, ongoing regulatory oversight will be essential to address emerging risks and ensure that e-liquids are manufactured to high standards.

USES

Since their introduction to the market around 2003, the use of e-cigarettes has surged rapidly. By 2011, approximately 7 million adults worldwide were using e-cigarettes, and this number skyrocketed to 68 million by 2020. In comparison, there were 1.1 billion cigarette smokers globally during the same period. The number of e-cigarette users continued to climb, reaching 82 million in 2021.

Several factors have contributed to this substantial increase in e-cigarette use. Targeted marketing campaigns have played a significant role, promoting e-cigarettes as a modern and safer alternative to traditional smoking. Additionally, e-cigarettes are generally more cost-effective than conventional cigarettes, making them an attractive option for many consumers. The perception of e-cigarettes as a safer option compared to tobacco has also driven their popularity, as users seek to reduce the health risks associated with smoking.

Geographically, the highest prevalence of e-cigarette use is observed in China, the United States, and Europe, with China leading in the number of users. This trend is likely influenced by factors such as market availability, regulatory environments, and cultural attitudes towards smoking and vaping in these regions.

The rapid rise in e-cigarette usage highlights the significant shift in consumer behavior and the growing preference for alternative nicotine delivery systems. As the market continues to expand, ongoing research and regulation will be essential to address the health implications and ensure the safe use of these products.

The reasons for e-cigarette use are diverse and multifaceted. A significant number of users turn to e-cigarettes as a means to quit smoking traditional tobacco products. This group often seeks a less harmful alternative to satisfy their nicotine cravings while attempting to reduce or eliminate their dependence on cigarettes.

However, not all e-cigarette use is driven by the desire to quit smoking. A substantial proportion of users engage in vaping for recreational purposes or to circumvent smoke-free laws that prohibit smoking in certain areas. These individuals may find vaping an enjoyable activity in its own right, separate from any smoking cessation efforts.

One of the primary motivations for many vapers is the belief that e-cigarettes are safer than traditional smoking. This perception is supported by various studies suggesting that vaping exposes users to fewer harmful chemicals compared to smoking combustible tobacco. The wide array of available flavors also plays a crucial role in attracting users, offering a customizable and enjoyable experience that traditional cigarettes cannot provide. Moreover, the lower cost of e-cigarettes compared to conventional cigarettes makes them a more economical choice for many consumers.

Additional motivations for using e-cigarettes include practical considerations such as the reduced odor and fewer stains associated with vaping. Unlike smoking, vaping produces a less intrusive scent and minimizes the staining of teeth and fingers, making it a more socially acceptable option in many settings.

E-cigarettes also hold particular appeal for technophiles who enjoy the opportunity to customize their devices. The ability to modify and personalize e-cigarette hardware and e-liquid formulations allows these users to enhance their vaping experience according to their preferences and technical interests.

In summary, the reasons for e-cigarette use are varied and encompass a range of practical, economic, and recreational factors. The desire to quit smoking, perceptions of safety, flavor variety, cost savings, and the appeal of reduced odor and stains all contribute to the popularity of e-cigarettes. Additionally, the customization aspect attracts a niche group of users who find enjoyment in personalizing their vaping devices.

The gateway hypothesis posits that the use of less harmful substances can lead to the consumption of more dangerous ones. This concept is often applied to e-cigarettes, suggesting that individuals who begin by vaping may eventually progress to smoking traditional cigarettes. Research supports this idea, indicating that many vapers also become smokers. This pattern is particularly pronounced among individuals with mental illnesses, who are generally more vulnerable to nicotine addiction and thus at a higher risk for dual use of vaping and smoking.

However, the observed association between vaping and subsequent smoking does not inherently confirm a causal gateway effect. Instead, it is possible that certain underlying characteristics predispose individuals to engage in both activities. For example, genetic factors have been linked to a range of risk-taking behaviors, including smoking, vaping, gambling, and promiscuity. Additionally, young people with poor executive functioning are more likely to use e-cigarettes, cigarettes, and alcohol at higher rates than their peers. E-cigarette users are also more prone to consuming marijuana and misusing prescription stimulants like Adderall or Ritalin.

Critics of longitudinal studies on e-cigarettes and smoking argue that these studies often fail to adequately account for various confounding factors, such as genetic predispositions and psychological traits, that could influence both vaping and smoking behaviors. Consequently, the evidence for a direct causal relationship between vaping and smoking remains inconclusive.

Despite the concerns raised by the gateway hypothesis, smoking rates have continued to decline as e-cigarette use has become more popular, particularly among young people. This trend suggests that there is little evidence to support the idea of a gateway effect at the population level. Nevertheless, some experts argue that this observation might overlook the impact of anti-smoking interventions and policies that have been implemented concurrently with the rise of e-cigarettes.

Overall, while the gateway hypothesis raises important questions about the potential risks of vaping, the evidence remains mixed. Further research is needed to disentangle the complex relationships between vaping, smoking, and other risk-taking behaviors, and to determine the true impact of e-cigarettes on public health.

Globally, an increasing number of young people are turning to e-cigarettes. This trend has been accompanied by a significant decline in tobacco use among youth, with estimates suggesting a reduction of about 75% in traditional cigarette smoking. Despite this positive trend, there are complexities in the patterns of e-cigarette use among young people.

Most young e-cigarette users have never smoked traditional cigarettes. However, there remains a notable minority who both vape and smoke, engaging in dual use. A considerable number of young people who would not typically smoke are now experimenting with vaping, often due to the appealing variety of flavors available in e-liquids. For many, the first experience with vaping involves a flavored product, which highlights the role that flavors play in attracting young users.

Additionally, young people who smoke tobacco or marijuana, or who consume alcohol, are significantly more likely to also vape. This correlation suggests that vaping is part of a broader pattern of risk-taking behaviors among youth. Despite the decline in smoking rates, vaping seems to correlate with smoking among young people, even among those who might otherwise be unlikely to pick up smoking.

Experimentation with vaping has been shown to encourage some young people to continue smoking. For instance, a 2015 study found that minors faced little resistance when attempting to purchase e-cigarettes online, highlighting a gap in regulatory enforcement. Furthermore, the actual prevalence of vaping among teenagers might be underreported due to the use of alternative terms like "hookah pen" and reluctance to admit e-cigarette use in surveys.

More recent studies have documented a rising trend in e-cigarette use among young people. In 2018, 20% of high school students in the United States reported using e-cigarettes. By 2020, this figure had surged to 50%, indicating a rapid increase in adoption rates. Similar trends have been observed in Canada, where the percentage of young people reporting e-cigarette use rose from 29% in 2017 to 37% in 2018.

These statistics underscore the growing popularity of e-cigarettes among youth and the need for continued monitoring and regulation to address this public health challenge. The increase in e-cigarette use among young people raises important questions about long-term health impacts and the effectiveness of current policies aimed at curbing youth vaping.

CHAPTER THREE

HEALTH EFFECTS

The health risks associated with e-cigarettes remain uncertain, but current evidence suggests that the likelihood of serious adverse events is relatively low. E-cigarettes are generally considered to be safer than traditional combusted tobacco products. However, this does not imply that they are without harm.

E-cigarette use has been linked to an increased risk of several respiratory conditions, including chronic obstructive pulmonary disease (COPD), asthma, chronic bronchitis, and emphysema. The risk is higher among individuals who use e-cigarettes daily compared to those who use them occasionally. According to the National Academies of Sciences, Engineering, and Medicine, laboratory tests of e-cigarette ingredients, in vitro toxicological tests, and short-term human studies suggest that e-cigarettes are likely to be significantly less harmful than combustible tobacco cigarettes.

Randomized controlled trials have provided strong evidence that e-cigarettes containing nicotine are more effective than nicotine replacement therapy (NRT) in helping people quit smoking. There is also moderate-certainty evidence indicating that nicotine-containing e-cigarettes are more effective than nicotine-free e-cigarettes for smoking cessation.

While serious adverse effects are rare, e-cigarette use can lead to less severe but still troubling symptoms such as abdominal pain, headaches, blurred vision, throat and mouth irritation, vomiting, nausea, and coughing. Nicotine, a common component of e-liquids, is addictive and poses specific risks to fetuses, children, and young people, potentially affecting brain development and overall health.

In 2019 and 2020, the United States experienced an outbreak of severe lung illnesses linked to vaping. The Centers for Disease Control and Prevention (CDC) identified vitamin E acetate, a substance sometimes used in vape liquids, as a potential cause of these illnesses. The precise cause of the outbreak is still debated, with vitamin E acetate being one of the identified culprits, but it is likely that multiple factors contributed to the health issues observed during this period.

Overall, while e-cigarettes may be a safer alternative to traditional smoking, they are not risk-free. Continued research and regulatory oversight are necessary to fully understand the health impacts of e-cigarette use and to ensure consumer safety.

E-cigarettes generate particulate matter at levels comparable to those produced by traditional tobacco cigarettes. Despite this similarity, there is only limited evidence demonstrating adverse respiratory and cardiovascular effects in humans. A 2020 review highlighted this gap in knowledge and emphasized the need for more long-term studies to comprehensively assess the health impacts of e-cigarette use.

Current research indicates that using e-cigarettes increases the risk of developing respiratory conditions. Specifically, e-cigarette use is associated with a 40% higher risk of asthma and a 50% higher risk of chronic obstructive pulmonary disease (COPD) compared to individuals who do not use nicotine products at all. These findings underscore the potential health risks posed by e-cigarettes, despite their reputation as a safer alternative to traditional smoking.

The particulate matter emitted by e-cigarettes can penetrate deep into the lungs, potentially leading to inflammation and other respiratory issues over time. The cardiovascular effects of e-cigarette use are also a growing concern, with initial studies suggesting potential impacts on heart health. However, the current body of evidence is insufficient to draw definitive conclusions, prompting calls for more rigorous and long-term research.

Understanding the full extent of the health risks associated with e-cigarettes is crucial, particularly as their popularity continues to rise. Regulatory bodies and public health organizations need comprehensive data to inform guidelines and policies that protect consumers. As e-cigarettes remain a relatively new product, ongoing research will be essential in determining their long-term safety and health implications.

In summary, while e-cigarettes produce particulate matter at levels similar to traditional cigarettes, the evidence of their adverse health effects is still limited. The increased risk of asthma and COPD associated with e-cigarette use highlights the need for caution and further study. Long-term research is necessary to fully understand the respiratory and cardiovascular impacts of e-cigarettes and to ensure that public health policies can adequately address these risks.

Pregnancy

The British Royal College of Midwives has stated that while vaping devices, such as electronic cigarettes (e-cigarettes), do contain some toxic substances, these are present at significantly lower levels compared to those found in tobacco smoke. The organization supports the use of e-cigarettes by pregnant women who are trying to quit smoking, noting that if an e-cigarette helps a smoker to cease smoking and maintain a smoke-free status, it should be endorsed. Furthermore, based on current evidence regarding e-cigarette safety, there is no indication that using an e-cigarette negatively affects breastfeeding. The Royal College of Midwives encourages continued use of e-cigarettes if they assist in quitting smoking and maintaining abstinence from tobacco.

Similarly, the UK National Health Service (NHS) has emphasized that if e-cigarettes aid in quitting smoking, they present a safer alternative for both the mother and her baby compared to continuing smoking. This guidance reflects the perception among many women that vaping is a safer option during pregnancy than smoking traditional tobacco.

Despite this, it is important to note that many women choose to vape during pregnancy due to the perceived safety benefits of e-cigarettes over conventional tobacco products. This ongoing use highlights the need for further research and continued public health support to ensure that pregnant women receive accurate information about the relative risks and benefits of e-cigarettes.

In a limited study conducted in 2015, which surveyed 316 pregnant women at a clinic in Maryland, it was found that a majority of participants were aware of e-cigarettes. Among them, 13% had used e-cigarettes at some point, and 0.6% were identified as daily users. These findings raise concerns as the nicotine delivery from e-cigarettes can be as high as or even exceed that of traditional cigarettes.

Further data from the Pregnancy Risk Assessment System (PRAMS), collected from two states, reveals that in 2015—around the midpoint of the study period—10.8% of women used e-cigarettes in the three months prior to pregnancy. The usage rates decreased over time, with 7.0% using e-cigarettes during pregnancy, 5.8% in the first trimester, and 1.4% at the time of birth. Additionally, data from the National Health

Interview Survey (NHIS) covering 2014 to 2017 indicate that 38.9% of pregnant smokers used e-cigarettes, compared to only 13.5% of smokers who were not pregnant but of reproductive age. A health economic study found that implementing a minimum legal sale age for e-cigarettes in the United States led to a 0.6 percentage point increase in teenage prenatal smoking, with no observed impact on birth outcomes. This underscores the need for further research into the health effects of e-cigarette use during pregnancy.

The Centers for Disease Control and Prevention (CDC) advises against the use of e-cigarettes during pregnancy. While e-cigarette aerosol generally contains fewer harmful substances compared to cigarette smoke, nicotine remains a significant health hazard. Nicotine can adversely affect both the health of pregnant women and the developing fetus, potentially impairing brain and lung development. Additionally, some of the flavorings used in e-cigarettes may pose risks to a developing baby.

In the realm of e-cigarette usage among youth, the Juul vaporizer gained substantial popularity until 2022, when the FDA imposed a sales ban on its products. A 2017 study by the Truth Initiative found that nearly 80% of respondents aged 15 to 24 who used Juul had used the device within the past 30 days. During the 2010s, the term "Juuling" became commonly used among American teenagers to describe vaping, and Juul-related content became a frequent subject of memes on social media platforms.

Harm Reduction

Harm reduction encompasses strategies aimed at reducing the adverse effects associated with a particular behavior from a prior level. Specifically, harm minimization focuses on mitigating risks to the lowest possible extent. In the context of nicotine use, harm minimization involves efforts to replace tobacco exposure with less harmful alternatives, such as e-cigarettes, for individuals who are unable or unwilling to quit nicotine entirely. E-cigarettes have the potential to lower smokers' exposure to carcinogens and other toxic substances present in traditional tobacco products.

The concept of tobacco harm reduction has sparked considerable debate within the field of tobacco control. Health advocates have been cautious in endorsing harm reduction approaches, largely due to concerns about the reliability of tobacco companies in producing safer products. The apprehension is that these companies may not be trustworthy in their efforts to reduce the risks associated with tobacco use. Despite this, a significant number of smokers are interested in utilizing e-cigarettes as a means to reduce harm from smoking.

However, the harm reduction argument does not fully address the negative effects of nicotine itself. There is considerable debate about the appropriateness of harm reduction strategies for children and adolescents who may use nicotine-containing e-cigarettes. Quitting smoking entirely is widely recognized as the most effective method for reducing tobacco-related harm.

Tobacco smoke is known to contain approximately 100 carcinogens and 900 additional chemicals with potential cancer-causing properties. In contrast, e-cigarette vapor has been shown to contain fewer carcinogens than tobacco smoke. A 2015 study using a third-generation e-cigarette device found that formaldehyde levels could exceed those found in cigarette smoke when the device was used at maximum power settings. This highlights that e-cigarettes cannot be deemed entirely safe, as no level of carcinogens is considered risk-free.

Given their resemblance to traditional cigarettes, e-cigarettes might serve a beneficial role in harm reduction efforts. However, the public health community remains divided on whether to endorse e-cigarettes as a viable option for smoking cessation, given the uncertainties surrounding their safety and efficacy. Overall, the evidence suggests a cautious approach to implementing harm reduction strategies that promote e-cigarettes as a safer alternative to smoking, while ensuring that protective measures are in place for vulnerable populations and individuals.

A primary concern regarding the use of e-cigarettes is the potential for smokers who might have quit entirely to develop an alternative nicotine addiction. The phenomenon of dual use, where individuals continue to smoke traditional cigarettes while also using e-cigarettes, may pose additional health risks. Even minimal use of conventional cigarettes alongside vaping could be detrimental, and the convenience of e-cigarettes might further increase the likelihood of ongoing nicotine dependence. The notion of promoting vaping as a harm reduction tool may be premature. A 2011 review suggested that e-cigarettes hold the potential to reduce tobacco-related mortality and morbidity. However, there remains a lack of definitive evidence to fully substantiate these claims, and the health benefits of combining cigarette reduction with e-cigarette use are not yet clear.

Despite the potential role e-cigarettes could play in tobacco harm reduction, there is caution against the possibility of overregulating these products. Such regulation might inadvertently limit their effectiveness as a smoking cessation aid. Health professionals are advised to carefully consider recommending e-cigarettes to smokers who are unwilling to quit through other means, as a potentially safer alternative to smoking.

A 2014 review suggested that e-cigarette regulations should be akin to those applied to dietary supplements or cosmetic products to avoid impeding their potential for harm reduction. Meanwhile, a 2012 review indicated that e-cigarettes could significantly reduce the use of traditional cigarettes and might serve as a lower-risk substitute, though insufficient data exists on their safety and efficacy to draw definitive conclusions. Additionally, there is a lack of research on the effectiveness of vaping in reducing harm for high-risk groups, such as individuals with mental health disorders.

The 2014 Public Health England (PHE) report concluded that the hazards associated with current e-cigarette products are likely minimal and substantially lower than those of smoking. Nonetheless, it suggested that further reductions in harm could be achieved through the establishment of reasonable product standards. The British Medical Association supports the use of conventional nicotine replacement therapies but acknowledges that, for patients who are unable or unwilling to use these methods, e-cigarettes may be a preferable alternative to traditional tobacco smoking.

The American Association of Public Health Physicians (AAPHP) advocates for considering other nicotine-containing products, such as e-cigarettes and smokeless tobacco, for individuals who are either unwilling or unable to quit smoking through medical or pharmaceutical methods. A 2014 World Health Organization (WHO) report found that while some smokers might transition completely to e-cigarettes from traditional tobacco, a significant number are likely to engage in dual use. The report highlighted that dual use would have substantially smaller benefits for overall survival compared to complete cessation of smoking.

Smoking Cessation

The effectiveness of e-cigarettes in aiding smoking cessation remains a topic of considerable debate. Current evidence, although limited, suggests that e-cigarettes may be beneficial in helping people quit smoking, particularly when used in clinical settings. However, the reality is that a significant number of users tend to become dual users, continuing to smoke traditional cigarettes while using e-cigarettes, rather than achieving complete abstinence. Outside of clinical environments, the impact of vaping on smoking cessation appears to be minimal.

Research into whether e-cigarettes can reduce the number of cigarettes smoked by individuals is sparse but suggests that e-cigarette use might decrease cigarette consumption. Nonetheless, even smoking a small number of cigarettes daily—ranging from one to four—can substantially increase the risk of cardiovascular disease compared to non-smoking. The relationship between reducing cigarette consumption through vaping and achieving full cessation remains unclear.

It is also uncertain whether e-cigarettes are equally effective for all types of smokers. While vaping with nicotine may aid in reducing tobacco use among daily smokers, its effectiveness as a smoking cessation tool may depend on whether it is part of a broader quit attempt.

A significant challenge in evaluating e-cigarettes is the sheer variety of brands, models, and liquid compositions available, coupled with ongoing technological advancements. Unlike nicotine replacement therapies, e-cigarettes have not undergone rigorous efficacy testing. Additionally, there are social considerations: e-cigarettes might normalize tobacco use and potentially extend cigarette use among individuals who might otherwise quit. Conversely, they could exert pressure on smokers to quit by presenting a more socially acceptable alternative. Evidence suggests that smokers are more likely to successfully quit using e-cigarettes with tank systems compared to cigalikes, possibly due to more effective nicotine delivery. Some studies also indicate that e-cigarettes may be preferred over other pharmaceutical options for smoking cessation.

The quality of evidence supporting the long-term effectiveness of vaping compared to nicotine-free e-cigarettes is low. Nicotine-containing e-cigarettes have been associated with greater success in smoking cessation than those without nicotine. A 2013 study found that vaping, with or without nicotine, reduced cigarette consumption among smokers not actively trying to quit. E-cigarettes without nicotine might help alleviate tobacco cravings due to their ability to replicate smoking-related physical stimuli.

A meta-analysis from 2015 revealed that nicotine-containing e-cigarettes are more effective for quitting smoking than nicotine-free versions, with 20% of users managing to quit compared to 10% with other nicotine replacement products. A 2016 review also noted a trend towards greater effectiveness of nicotine-containing e-cigarettes for smoking cessation, though the evidence was not robust. The impact of flavored e-cigarettes on quitting remains inconclusive, and there is tentative evidence suggesting that health warnings on vaping products may encourage users to quit vaping.

As of 2020, the efficacy and safety of vaping for smoking cessation during pregnancy remain unknown, with no specific research available on this topic. Evidence strongly suggests that vaping is not effective for smoking cessation among adolescents. Given the current evidence gaps, vaping is not recommended for cancer patients, although it is generally considered less harmful than smoking cigarettes. The effectiveness of vaping as a smoking cessation tool for vulnerable groups remains uncertain.

Safety

The risks associated with e-cigarette use are the subject of considerable debate and lack a clear consensus. Despite the growing prevalence of e-cigarettes, comprehensive safety data is still limited. This is partly due to the wide variety of e-liquid formulations, each with different components that are present in the aerosol inhaled by users. Reviews on the safety of e-cigarettes have produced diverse findings, reflecting the complexity of assessing their risks.

A 2014 report by the World Health Organization (WHO) highlighted potential risks related to e-cigarette use, cautioning that their long-term safety remains uncertain. While products regulated by the U.S. Food and Drug Administration (FDA), such as nicotine inhalers, might be considered safer alternatives, e-cigarettes are generally perceived as less hazardous compared to traditional tobacco products like cigarettes and cigars.

The risk of early death associated with e-cigarettes is expected to be comparable to that of smokeless tobacco products. Since e-cigarettes do not involve combustion and do not contain tobacco, users potentially avoid several harmful substances typically found in tobacco smoke, such as ash, tar, and carbon monoxide. However, e-cigarette use, whether or not it includes nicotine, cannot be deemed entirely risk-free due to the unknown long-term effects of their use. The absence of combustion and tobacco does not fully eliminate the potential risks associated with e-cigarettes.

The cytotoxicity of e-liquids used in e-cigarettes can vary significantly, and contamination by various chemicals has been identified in these liquids. For instance, metal components within e-cigarettes, such as those in the heating elements, can introduce metal particles into the e-liquid. When the nichrome wire (a common heating element) heats up and interacts with the e-liquid, it can inadvertently produce carbonyl compounds, including formaldehyde. Although typical e-cigarette usage and devices operating at reduced voltages (around 3.0 V) produce minimal levels of formaldehyde, later-generation and "tank-style" e-cigarettes that operate at higher voltages (approximately 5.0 V) have the potential to generate formaldehyde levels comparable to or even exceeding those found in traditional cigarette smoke.

A 2015 report by Public Health England noted that high levels of formaldehyde were mainly produced during "dry-puffing" or overheating, which is usually detected and avoided by users. The report concluded that there was no substantial evidence indicating that e-cigarette users are exposed to dangerously high levels of aldehydes. Nonetheless, users might develop a tolerance to the unpleasant taste caused by elevated aldehyde levels, especially when nicotine cravings are strong.

Another chemical commonly found in e-cigarettes is ketene. When inhaled, ketene can damage lung tissue cells, impairing their function and gas absorption capabilities. This can result in shortness of breath and potentially lead to more severe health issues such as tachycardia and respiratory failure. Users of nicotine-containing e-cigarettes are exposed to the associated risks of nicotine, including cardiovascular disease, potential birth defects, and poisoning. Although nicotine has been linked to cancer in laboratory studies, there is insufficient evidence to confirm its carcinogenicity in humans. The long-term health impacts of inhaling propylene glycol, glycerin, and flavorings in e-cigarette vapor are not well understood.

In October 2021, research conducted by Johns Hopkins University identified over 2,000 unknown chemicals in the vapor produced by popular e-cigarette brands such as Vuse, Juul, Blu, and Mi-Salt. Additionally, a vaping-related lung illness outbreak in the US and Canada during 2019–2020 was primarily associated with the use of THC-containing products mixed with vitamin E acetate.

E-cigarettes generate vapor composed of fine and ultrafine particulate matter, with a significant proportion of these particles falling into the ultrafine category. The vapor contains a range of substances, including propylene glycol, glycerin, nicotine, flavorings, small amounts of toxicants, carcinogens, and heavy metals, as well as metal nanoparticles. Carcinogenic compounds such as N-Nitrosonornicotine (NNN) and N-Nitrosoanatabine (NAT) have been detected in e-cigarettes, with known harmful effects on human health. The composition of the vapor can vary greatly depending on the e-liquid's ingredients, the device's design and operation, and user behavior.

E-cigarette vapor may contain potentially harmful chemicals not present in traditional tobacco smoke. Although the majority of toxic substances found in cigarette smoke are absent in e-cigarette vapor, the vapor still contains lower concentrations of some potentially hazardous chemicals compared to cigarette smoke. The levels of these chemicals are typically well below 1% of the limits established by workplace safety standards. However, it is important to note that these standards do not account for specific vulnerable groups, such as individuals with medical conditions, children, or infants, who might be exposed to second-hand vapor.

There are concerns about the potential health risks associated with inhaling mainstream vapor exhaled by e-cigarette users, especially in enclosed spaces. Despite the fact that pollutant levels in e-cigarette vapor are significantly lower than those in cigarette smoke, and the risks are considered to be much lower, there is still apprehension about potential health impacts. Additionally, there is a worry that e-cigarette use by parents could inadvertently expose their children to harmful substances.

A review conducted in 2014 suggested that e-cigarettes should be regulated to ensure consumer safety. There is also limited research on the environmental impact of e-cigarettes, particularly concerning the production, use, and disposal of cartridge-based devices. Non-reusable e-cigarettes could contribute to the growing issue of electronic waste, posing additional environmental concerns.

Addiction

Nicotine, a principal component in most e-liquids, is widely recognized for its high addictive potential, comparable to substances such as heroin and cocaine. This substance is known to induce addiction through complex mechanisms associated with brain plasticity, which is the brain's ability to reorganize itself based on experiences. The reinforcing effects of nicotine significantly contribute to both the initiation and maintenance of its use. Approximately 32% of individuals who use nicotine for the first time develop a dependence on it.

The process of nicotine addiction encompasses both psychological and physical aspects of dependence. Nicotine-containing e-cigarette vapor induces changes in neurochemical, physiological, and behavioral processes related to addiction. This substance impacts a wide array of bodily systems, including neurological, neuromuscular, cardiovascular, respiratory, immunological, and gastrointestinal systems.

Long-term use of nicotine leads to neuroplastic changes within the brain's reward system, resulting in nicotine dependence. The neurophysiological mechanisms underlying this dependence are complex and influenced by genetic factors, age, gender, and environmental conditions. Nicotine addiction alters several neural systems, including dopaminergic, glutamatergic, GABAergic, and serotoninergic pathways, which are involved in the body's response to nicotine.

Extended nicotine use also affects a broad spectrum of genes related to neurotransmission, signal transduction, and synaptic structure. Genetic factors play a significant role in an individual's ability to quit smoking, including variations in how nicotine is metabolized. This highlights the intricate relationship between genetic predispositions and the challenges of overcoming nicotine addiction.

Nicotine, a parasympathomimetic stimulant, functions by binding to and activating nicotinic acetylcholine receptors in the brain. This activation triggers the release of various neurotransmitters, including dopamine, norepinephrine, acetylcholine, serotonin, gamma-aminobutyric acid, glutamate, and endorphins. Additionally, several neuropeptides such as proopiomelanocortin-derived α-MSH and adrenocorticotropic hormone are also released. Key players in nicotine addiction include corticotropin-releasing factor, neuropeptide Y, orexins, and norepinephrine. Chronic nicotine exposure can lead to an increase in the number of nicotinic receptors, a process believed to result from receptor desensitization followed by receptor upregulation.

Extended nicotine exposure can lead to a downregulation of glutamate transporter 1 and alterations in receptor activity, specifically upregulating cortical nicotinic receptors while reducing their activity in cortical vasodilation regions. These neuroadaptive changes are complex and not fully understood. Tolerance to nicotine develops over time, partly due to the creation of new nicotinic acetylcholine receptors in the brain.

After several months of abstinence from nicotine, receptor levels typically return to baseline. However, the full extent of the reversibility of brain alterations caused by nicotine is not entirely clear. Nicotine also stimulates nicotinic acetylcholine receptors in the adrenal medulla, leading to elevated levels of epinephrine and beta-endorphin. These effects are a result of nicotine's stimulation of nicotinic acetylcholine receptors, which are present throughout both the central and peripheral nervous systems.

Upon cessation of nicotine intake, the upregulated nicotinic acetylcholine receptors can induce withdrawal symptoms. These symptoms may include cravings for nicotine, irritability, anxiety, depression, impatience, sleep disturbances, restlessness, increased hunger, weight gain, and difficulty concentrating. When attempting to quit smoking through vaping with a nicotine-containing base, individuals may experience withdrawal symptoms similar to those mentioned. The neurobiological changes induced by nicotine lead to a sense of abnormality when nicotine is not present, compelling users to maintain nicotine intake to achieve a sense of normalcy. E-cigarettes might mitigate cigarette cravings and withdrawal symptoms to some extent, but their effectiveness varies.

The impact of e-cigarette use on overall nicotine addiction remains uncertain. Although the nicotine content in e-cigarettes is sufficient to sustain dependence, the effect of e-cigarettes on addiction levels is not fully understood. Chronic nicotine exposure leads to significant neuroplastic adaptations in the brain, making cessation difficult. A 2015 study highlighted that users of non-nicotine e-liquids still exhibited signs of dependence, indicating that the experience of vaping alone can contribute to addictive behaviors. Experienced vapers may take longer puffs, potentially leading to increased nicotine intake. Assessing the full impact of e-cigarette use on nicotine dependence is challenging due to the diverse range of e-cigarette products available. As these devices have evolved, they have improved their efficiency in delivering nicotine, which could potentially enhance their addiction potential.

In a 2015 policy statement, the American Academy of Pediatrics (AAP) expressed concern about the potential for e-cigarettes to create a new generation of nicotine-dependent youth, potentially reversing decades of progress in tobacco control. Similarly, the World Health Organization (WHO) has raised alarms about initiating nicotine use among non-smokers, and the National Institute on Drug Abuse has noted that e-cigarettes might perpetuate nicotine addiction in those trying to quit. While the data available suggests that excessive use of e-cigarettes may be less common than with traditional cigarettes, there is a lack of long-term studies on their effectiveness in treating tobacco addiction. Evidence indicates that dual use of e-cigarettes and traditional cigarettes might be associated with higher levels of nicotine dependence.

There is growing concern that children who start with vaping may eventually progress to smoking. Adolescents, who often underestimate nicotine's addictiveness, may be particularly vulnerable to developing a lifelong addiction due to their brain's heightened sensitivity to nicotine's effects. Minimal exposure to nicotine during adolescence can potentially lead to significant neuroplastic changes in the brain. A 2014 review revealed that a significant portion of young people who had never tried traditional cigarettes had used e-cigarettes. However, it is unclear to what extent teenagers may be using e-cigarettes in unintended ways, such as increasing nicotine delivery, and how this usage might contribute to addiction or substance dependence.

The debate surrounding e-cigarette legislation is influenced by their overlap with existing tobacco laws and medical drug policies, and is ongoing in many countries. In May 2016, the European Union implemented the revised Tobacco Products Directive, which introduced stricter regulations for e-cigarettes. In the United States, the legal status of e-cigarettes has evolved over time; in February 2010, the US District Court ruled against the FDA's attempt to classify e-cigarettes as "drug-devices," and by December 2010, the US Court of Appeals confirmed that e-cigarettes should be regulated as tobacco products under the Family Smoking Prevention and Tobacco Control Act of 2009. In August 2016, the US FDA expanded its regulatory authority to include e-cigarettes, cigars, and other tobacco products. As a result, large tobacco companies have significantly ramped up their marketing efforts for these products.

In both the US and Europe, the scientific community is primarily concerned with the potential public health implications of e-cigarettes. Public health experts are wary that e-cigarettes might normalize smoking, undermine existing tobacco control measures, and potentially act as a gateway to smoking among youth. The public health community remains divided on whether to endorse e-cigarettes, given the uncertainties regarding their safety and efficacy in smoking cessation. While there is acknowledgment of the potential benefits of e-cigarettes in quitting smoking and reducing harm, concerns persist about their long-term safety and the risk of creating a new generation of nicotine-dependent users. Tobacco control advocates worry that widespread use of e-cigarettes could introduce its own set of health risks similar to those of tobacco smoking due to chronic exposure.

Medical organizations hold varying opinions on the health effects of vaping. There is a consensus that e-cigarettes generally expose users to fewer toxic substances compared to traditional tobacco cigarettes. However, some healthcare groups and policymakers are cautious about recommending e-cigarettes as a smoking cessation tool due to the limited evidence regarding their effectiveness and safety. Proposals range from banning e-cigarette sales to regulating them as tobacco products with reduced nicotine content or even as medicinal products.

A 2019 report by the World Health Organization (WHO) concluded that the available scientific evidence does not substantiate the tobacco industry's claims that e-cigarettes are less harmful than conventional tobacco products. Furthermore, the report highlighted a lack of sufficient evidence to support the use of e-cigarettes as an effective tool for smoking cessation. In contrast, healthcare organizations in the United Kingdom, including the Royal College of Physicians and Public Health England, have recommended that smokers consider switching to e-cigarettes or other nicotine replacement therapies if they are unable to quit smoking entirely. This recommendation is based on the potential for e-cigarettes to contribute to significant public health benefits and potentially save millions of lives.

On the other hand, major health organizations in the United States, such as the American Cancer Society, the American Heart Association, and the Surgeon General, have issued warnings regarding the potential negative impacts of e-cigarettes on cardiovascular and pulmonary health. They stress that the current evidence does not sufficiently demonstrate the safety and efficacy of e-cigarettes as a smoking cessation aid, advising caution until more robust evidence is available.

In 2016, the U.S. Food and Drug Administration (FDA) acknowledged that while electronic nicotine delivery systems (ENDS) might offer cessation benefits for individual smokers, none have been formally approved as effective smoking cessation aids. Similarly, in 2019, the European Respiratory Society expressed concerns about the long-term effects of e-cigarette use, noting that there is no evidence to suggest that e-cigarettes are safer than tobacco in the long term. The Society criticized the tobacco harm reduction strategy as being based on potentially incorrect or undocumented claims.

The Centers for Disease Control and Prevention (CDC) issued a precautionary statement on September 6, 2019, advising individuals to avoid using vaping products while the agency investigates numerous cases of severe lung illness and confirmed deaths linked to vaping in the United States. This ongoing investigation underscores the need for further research to clarify the risks associated with e-cigarette use.

SOCIETY AND CULTURE

Consumers have demonstrated a high level of enthusiasm and support for e-cigarettes, a level of engagement not seen with other nicotine replacement products. This widespread appeal positions e-cigarettes as a significant competitor to traditional combustible tobacco products.

By 2013, a distinct subculture known as "the vaping community" had emerged, with many members perceiving e-cigarettes as a safer alternative to smoking. For some, vaping has evolved into a hobby. Early online forums such as E-Cig-Reviews.com played a crucial role in fostering this community, and sites like UKVaper.org became hubs for discussing the practice of "modding," or customizing e-cigarette devices. The community also extends to social media platforms, including

Facebook and Reddit, where discussions and exchanges about vaping continue to flourish.

Vapers are actively involved in promoting their cause and often advocate for the benefits of e-cigarettes. Many e-cigarette companies maintain a robust online presence, supported by numerous vapers who write blogs and share their experiences on platforms like Twitter. A 2014 editorial in the Postgraduate Medical Journal noted that some vapers engage in highly aggressive online behavior toward those who criticize e-cigarettes, viewing them as a groundbreaking innovation with minimal risks.

A significant aspect of vaping culture includes a strong disdain for traditional tobacco companies. A 2014 review indicated that both tobacco and e-cigarette companies use consumer engagement to influence policy and oppose legislation that seeks to regulate e-cigarettes similarly to tobacco products. This strategy mirrors tactics used by the tobacco industry since the 1980s. In Europe, these methods were employed to mitigate the impact of the EU Tobacco Products Directive in October 2013. Grassroots lobbying also played a role in shaping the decision-making process regarding tobacco regulations. Additionally, tobacco companies have collaborated with organizations designed to promote e-cigarette use and have worked to undermine legislation aimed at restricting e-cigarette usage.

Large gatherings of vapers, known as vape meets, are held across the United States, bringing together enthusiasts to explore e-cigarette devices, accessories, and the associated lifestyle. These events provide a platform for attendees to engage with a wide range of specialized products and innovations not typically available at convenience stores or gas stations. Instead, many of these products are found online or at dedicated vape shops, where mainstream brands from large tobacco companies are less prevalent.

One notable event is Vapefest, which has been held annually since 2010 in various cities across the country. At these gatherings, participants often use and showcase community-created products and enjoy a range of activities related to vaping. Similarly, the Electronic Cigarette Convention, which began in 2013, serves as an annual meeting point for both companies and consumers to discuss and explore vaping innovations.

Some vapers engage in a practice known as "cloud-chasing," where they configure their atomizers to produce large volumes of vapor using low-resistance heating coils. This technique can place significant stress on the batteries, potentially leading to safety risks such as dangerous battery failures. Concerns have been raised within the vaping community about cloud-chasing, particularly regarding its impact on the public perception of vaping. Critics argue that this practice may contribute to a negative reputation for vapers when done in public spaces.

In 2014, the term "vape" was recognized as the Oxford Dictionaries' word of the year, reflecting the growing prominence and influence of vaping culture.

Regulations

Regulation of e-cigarettes differs significantly across various countries and regions, with some places imposing no regulations at all while others have enacted complete bans. For instance, in Japan, e-cigarettes containing nicotine are prohibited, resulting in the market primarily offering heated tobacco products as alternatives to traditional cigarettes. In contrast, other regions have implemented strict regulatory measures, with some even classifying e-cigarettes as medicinal products, as seen in the UK. However, as of February 2018, no e-cigarette device had been granted a medical license for commercial sale or prescription use in the UK. By 2015, approximately two-thirds of major nations had introduced some form of regulation for e-cigarettes.

The regulatory landscape for e-cigarettes is influenced by their intersection with tobacco laws and medical drug policies, prompting ongoing debates in many countries. E-cigarette manufacturers have actively lobbied for favorable legislation to support their interests. In 2016, the US Department of Transportation implemented a ban on the use of e-cigarettes on commercial flights, a regulation that applies to all flights to and from the United States. In 2018, the Royal College of Physicians called for a regulatory balance that ensures e-cigarette safety while encouraging smokers to switch from tobacco, and also for vigilance regarding any adverse effects that may arise.

Many countries are still in the process of determining the legal status of e-cigarettes. For example, e-cigarettes are banned in Brazil, Singapore, Uruguay, and India. In Canada, although nicotine-containing e-cigarettes were technically illegal to sell nationwide in 2014 due to the lack of regulation by Health Canada, this restriction is rarely enforced, and such products remain widely available. In 2016, Health Canada announced plans to introduce regulations for vaping products. In the United States and the United Kingdom, the sale and use of e-cigarettes by adults are legal. The revised EU Tobacco Products Directive, effective from May 2016, established stricter regulations for e-cigarettes, including limitations on advertising, restrictions on nicotine levels, and reduced use of flavors. While the directive does not prohibit vaping in public places, it mandates that purchasers of e-cigarettes be at least 18 years old. The updated directive has faced criticism from tobacco lobbyists concerned about its potential impact on their businesses.

As of August 8, 2016, the U.S. Food and Drug Administration (FDA) expanded its regulatory authority to encompass e-cigarettes, e-liquids, and all related products. This ruling requires the FDA to assess various aspects of these products, including their ingredients, features, health risks, and their appeal to minors and non-users. The new regulations also prohibit sales of e-cigarettes to individuals under 18, mandate photo identification for purchases, and ban their sale in vending machines accessible to all ages. Compliance deadlines for premarket review requirements for most e-cigarette and e-liquid products, initially set for November 2017, have been extended to August 8, 2022. This extension has led to legal challenges from organizations such as the American Heart Association, the American Academy of Pediatrics, and the Campaign for Tobacco-Free Kids.

In May 2016, under the authority of the Family Smoking Prevention and Tobacco Control Act, the FDA classified e-cigarette devices and e-liquids as tobacco products. This classification means that the FDA is responsible for regulating their marketing, labeling, and manufacturing processes. Vape shops that mix e-liquids or produce or modify devices are considered manufacturing sites and must register with the FDA and adhere to good manufacturing practices. In response, e-cigarette and tobacco companies have hired lobbyists to influence the FDA's regulatory actions and prevent the banning or restrictive evaluation of e-cigarette products.

In February 2014, the European Parliament enacted regulations requiring standardization and quality control for e-liquids and vaporizers, including ingredient disclosure and child-proof and tamper-proof packaging. The U.S. FDA proposed regulations for e-cigarettes in April 2014. Some U.S. states tax e-cigarettes as tobacco products, and many have expanded indoor smoking bans to include e-cigarettes. By April 2017, twelve U.S. states and 615 localities had banned e-cigarette use in places where traditional cigarette smoking is prohibited. Additionally, as of 2015, at least 48 states and two territories had banned e-cigarette sales to minors.

In November 2020, the New Zealand government introduced new vaping regulations requiring vape stores to register as specialist retailers to sell e-cigarettes, a broad range of flavored e-liquids, and other related products. These regulations mandate that vaping products be notified to the government before sale to ensure compliance with safety requirements and to verify that the ingredients do not contain prohibited substances.

In various countries, e-cigarettes containing nicotine have been classified as drug delivery devices, leading to restrictions or suspensions on their marketing until comprehensive safety and efficacy clinical trials are completed. Although e-cigarettes do not contain tobacco, their television advertising is not restricted in the U.S. Some nations have regulated e-cigarettes as medical products, despite not approving them as smoking cessation aids. A 2014 review highlighted growing concerns among health professionals, governments, and the public regarding e-cigarettes, recommending stringent regulation to protect consumers while noting that excessive regulation might inadvertently promote continued tobacco use. The review also suggested that regulation should be informed by documented adverse health effects.

Criticism of Vaping Bans

Critics of vaping bans argue that e-cigarettes are a significantly safer alternative to traditional tobacco products and that such bans may inadvertently drive individuals back to smoking combustible cigarettes. For instance, a 2015 article in the British Journal of Family Medicine claimed that e-cigarettes are up to 95% safer than conventional smoking. Furthermore, Ted Egan, San Francisco's chief economist, expressed concerns that the city's ban on e-cigarette sales could lead to an increase in cigarette smoking, as individuals who previously vaped might revert to traditional cigarettes. Critics argue that it is illogical to prohibit the sale of a safer alternative while allowing the continued sale of more harmful tobacco products. They emphasize that the objective should not be to criminalize tobacco use but to offer consumers the freedom to choose among available products.

In 2022, following an extensive review process, the U.S. Food and Drug Administration (FDA) denied Juul's application to continue selling its tobacco and menthol flavored vaping products. Opponents of this decision point to research published in

Nicotine and Tobacco Research, which indicated that smokers in North America who used Juul products were significantly more likely to switch to vaping compared to those in the United Kingdom who had access only to lower-strength nicotine products. Critics also highlight that the Biden administration's push to mandate lower-nicotine cigarettes overlooks the fact that nicotine alone is not the primary factor making cigarettes hazardous. They argue that vaping, which avoids many of the harmful components of combustible tobacco, such as the combustion process and various toxic chemicals, offers a safer alternative for those trying to quit smoking.

Product Liability

Numerous reports from the U.S. Fire Administration highlight incidents of electronic cigarettes causing fires and injuries to users and their surroundings. These issues are largely attributed to the design of the e-cigarettes, where the cartridges containing the liquid mixture are positioned dangerously close to the battery. According to a research report by the U.S. Fire Administration, this design flaw is exacerbated by the lack of protective measures for lithium-ion batteries used in some e-cigarettes, which can result in overheating of the coil.

In a 2015 report, the U.S. Fire Administration pointed out that electronic cigarettes are predominantly manufactured by independent factories rather than established tobacco companies. This lack of involvement from major tobacco firms often results in lower quality control standards during production. Consequently, the insufficient quality control has led to a number of incidents where e-cigarettes have caused injuries to individuals or damage to their surroundings.

Marketing

E-cigarettes are widely marketed as a safer alternative to traditional cigarettes, targeting a broad demographic that includes men, women, and children. They are also promoted to non-smokers, reflecting the extensive nature of e-cigarette advertising campaigns. There is increasing concern that these marketing efforts disproportionately target young adults, adolescents, and women. Major tobacco companies have significantly ramped up their marketing activities, raising the possibility that such strategies may not only expand e-cigarette use but also contribute to the re-glamorization of smoking. Some critics worry that e-cigarette advertising may intentionally or unintentionally promote smoking habits. A 2014 review noted that e-cigarette marketing has adopted aggressive techniques reminiscent of those used in cigarette advertising during the 1950s and 1960s.

E-cigarette companies are employing marketing strategies that echo those historically used by the tobacco industry to attract young consumers. These strategies are designed to cultivate a vaping culture that appeals to non-smokers, using themes and imagery similar to traditional cigarette advertisements, such as sexual content and customer satisfaction. A 2017 review observed that the tobacco industry envisions a future where e-cigarettes complement, rather than replace, tobacco use, with a particular focus on youth. E-cigarettes and nicotine are often portrayed as safe or even beneficial in media and on brand websites, raising further concerns.

While many countries have banned tobacco advertising, e-cigarette ads are still prevalent across various media platforms, including television, radio, magazines, newspapers, online channels, and retail stores. Between 2010 and 2014, e-cigarettes were the second most advertised product in magazines, trailing only behind traditional cigarettes. The acquisition of major e-cigarette brands by cigarette companies has enabled these firms to benefit from both the smoking and e-cigarette markets, while presenting themselves as champions of harm reduction. This dual market presence raises questions about the legitimacy of endorsing products that financially benefit the tobacco industry. Despite claims of supporting harm reduction, there is no evidence that these companies are phasing out traditional cigarettes. Moreover, advertising campaigns promoting e-cigarettes as smoking cessation tools in the US, UK, and China have not been endorsed by regulatory bodies.

In the United States, six leading e-cigarette companies spent $59.3 million on advertising in 2013. In both the US and Canada, over $2 million is annually allocated to online e-cigarette promotion. In 2012, many e-cigarette websites made unverified health claims, and the ease with which underage individuals could bypass age verification systems on these sites was a concern. About half of e-cigarette company websites included age restriction notices, although these measures were not always effective in preventing underage access and exposure to marketing.

Celebrity endorsements are frequently employed to promote e-cigarettes. For instance, a prominent 2012 US television advertising campaign featured actor Stephen Dorff, who was shown exhaling a substantial "cloud" of what the ad referred to as "vapor, not tobacco smoke." The campaign's message, directed at smokers, was framed as a call to reclaim personal freedom with the slogan, "We are all adults here, it's time to take our freedom back."

Critics of the tobacco industry argue that this marketing strategy mirrors tactics historically used to entice Americans into cigarette addiction. They contend that the Blu advertisement, set against a backdrop of a long-standing ban on tobacco advertising on television, reflects an effort to revive old norms that portray smoking as glamorous and socially acceptable. Cynthia Hallett of Americans for Non-Smokers' Rights criticized the campaign as an attempt to re-normalize smoking.

Joseph Cappella, a communications professor at the University of Pennsylvania, suggested that the advertisement's ocean setting was deliberately chosen to evoke an association between the e-cigarette and the concept of clean air. During 2012 and 2013, e-cigarette advertisements reached a significant television audience in the US, including 24 million young viewers. Channels such as AMC, Country Music Television, Comedy Central, WGN America, TV Land, and VH1 were particularly notable for attracting large numbers of young people aged 12 to 17.

Since at least 2007, e-cigarettes have been extensively advertised across global media platforms. These products are promoted vigorously, primarily through the Internet, as a safer alternative to traditional cigarettes. E-cigarette companies leverage social media platforms such as Facebook, Instagram, YouTube, and Twitter to market their products. High-profile endorsements include collaborations with celebrities and influencers from the sports and music industries. These campaigns often feature youthful and appealing imagery, including sexual content and music, and use slogans encouraging users to "take their freedom back."

Tobacco companies have aggressively targeted young audiences with e-cigarettes, employing marketing strategies that include cartoon characters and candy-flavored e-liquids. Social media is particularly rife with promotions for fruit-flavored e-liquids, which are among the most commonly advertised flavors.

Despite claims from e-cigarette companies that their products contain only water, nicotine, glycerin, propylene glycol, and flavorings, this representation is misleading. Research has revealed the presence of various heavy metals in e-cigarette vapor, including chromium, nickel, tin, silver, cadmium, mercury, and aluminum. The frequent assertion that e-cigarettes emit "only water vapor" is inaccurate; evidence shows that e-cigarette vapor contains potentially harmful chemicals such as nicotine, carbonyls, metals, volatile organic compounds, and particulate matter. This extensive advertising has also suggested that e-cigarettes pose minimal risk to non-users. However, numerous studies have documented adverse effects of secondhand vapor and shown that e-cigarettes can degrade indoor air quality.

Many e-cigarette companies promote their products as aids for smoking cessation, despite a lack of supporting evidence for their effectiveness. The marketing often includes unsubstantiated health claims, such as the assertion that e-cigarettes help with smoking cessation or improve psychiatric symptoms. These claims may particularly appeal to smokers with mental health issues. Additionally, e-cigarette advertising frequently highlights weight control benefits and promotes nicotine use with various flavors, which could attract specific demographics such as young people and those concerned about weight. Some companies also market their products as environmentally friendly without providing substantial evidence, which may be a tactic to boost sales.

Economics

From 2003 to 2014, there was a steady annual increase in e-cigarette sales. However, in 2015, the growth rate in e-cigarette usage in the United States experienced a slowdown. By January 2018, the expansion of e-cigarette usage in the UK had also diminished since 2013. In 2014, there were at least 466 distinct e-cigarette brands available on the market. Globally, e-cigarette sales reached approximately $7 billion in 2014 and grew to about $19.3 billion by 2019. Projections suggest that e-cigarette sales could potentially surpass traditional cigarette sales by 2023. Online sales account for roughly 30–50% of the total e-cigarette market. Established tobacco companies have secured a considerable portion of the e-cigarette market share.

As of 2018, approximately 95% of e-cigarette devices were manufactured in China, predominantly in the city of Shenzhen. Despite this, Chinese companies hold a relatively small market share in e-liquid sales. The rise in both online and offline sales of e-cigarettes began in 2014. In China, where combustible cigarettes are relatively inexpensive, the lower price of e-cigarettes may not significantly influence consumer preferences.

In 2015, tobacco companies were responsible for 80% of e-cigarette sales in convenience stores across the US. According to Nielsen Holdings, sales of e-cigarettes in convenience stores in the US declined for the first time during the four-week period ending May 10, 2014. This drop has been attributed to a shift in consumer behavior towards more specialized devices, referred to as "vapors-tanks-mods (VTMs)," which were not tracked by Nielsen. VTMs were estimated to constitute 57% of the $3.5 billion US market for vapor products in 2015.

In 2014, dollar sales of customizable e-cigarettes and e-liquids surpassed those of cigalikes in the US, despite customizable options generally being less expensive. The Smoke-Free Alternatives Trade Association estimated that there were 35,000 vape shops in the US in 2014, a significant increase from the previous year. However, the slowdown in market growth in 2015 also impacted the VTMs segment.

Major tobacco retailers continue to dominate the cigalike market. In April 2018, Jim Cramer of Mad Money remarked on the dramatic impact that the rise of vaping had on traditional cigarette manufacturers, noting how the recognition of this disruption led to a sharp decline in tobacco stocks. In 2019, a vaping industry organization warned that a potential US ban on e-cigarette flavors could have significant repercussions, potentially affecting over 150,000 jobs across the country.

In the United States, the dominant player in the e-cigarette market is Juul, which was launched in June 2015. As of August 2018, Juul held a commanding 72% share of the US e-cigarette market, according to Nielsen data. In contrast, its nearest competitor, RJ Reynolds' Vuse, captured less than 10% of the market. Juul's rapid rise in popularity was notable, with its market share increasing by 700% in just 2016. In response to Juul's success, RJ Reynolds announced on July 17, 2018, that it would introduce a pod mod device similar to Juul in August 2018. The success of Juul has spurred a surge of similar pod devices entering the market.

In Canada, the e-cigarette market was valued at approximately 140 million CAD in 2015. There is a growing presence of e-cigarette retail outlets across the country. A 2014 audit revealed that 94% of grocery stores, convenience stores, and tobacconist shops in four Canadian cities only sold nicotine-free e-cigarettes, whereas all vape shops offered at least one nicotine-containing product.

By 2015, the e-cigarette market in the UK had reached only about 5% of the size of the tobacco market. In that year, the leading cigalike brands were largely owned by tobacco companies, though most tank-type e-cigarettes were produced by non-tobacco industry firms. Some products from the tobacco industry, despite using prefilled cartridges, were designed to resemble tank models.

In France, Groupe Xerfi estimated the e-cigarette market to be valued at €130 million in 2015, with the e-liquid market reaching €265 million. As of December 2015, there were 2,400 vape shops in France, a decrease of 400 from March of the same year. Industry group Fivape attributed this reduction to consolidation within the sector rather than decreased demand.

Vietnam's e-cigarette market is expanding rapidly, with usage rates increasing 18-fold from 2015 to 2020. Among adolescents aged 13 to 15, e-cigarette use rose to 3.5% by 2020, up 1.6% from 2019. The World Health Organization (WHO) estimates global economic losses from tobacco to be $1.4 trillion annually, accounting for about 1% of global GDP. In Vietnam, efforts are underway to regulate the e-cigarette market; however, challenges persist, including limited public awareness of the potential harms of e-cigarettes, unclear legal frameworks, and intense competition from imported e-cigarette products.

ENVIRONMENTAL IMPACT

Reusable e-cigarettes present a significant advantage over traditional cigarettes in terms of waste reduction. Unlike conventional cigarettes, which generate litter in the form of discarded butts that often end up polluting oceans, reusable e-cigarettes do not produce such waste after each use. Traditional cigarette butts, though they do eventually undergo biodegradation and photodegradation, still contribute to environmental pollution. Some e-cigarette brands have initiated recycling programs for their cartridges and batteries, but the extent and effectiveness of these recycling efforts remain unclear.

However, non-reusable e-cigarettes contribute to the growing issue of electronic waste. Improper disposal of these products can result in the release of hazardous materials, including heavy metals, nicotine, and other chemicals from batteries and residual e-liquid. A study conducted between July 2018 and April 2019 found that e-cigarette products accounted for 19% of the waste collected from traditional and electronic tobacco and cannabis products at 12 public high schools in Northern California.

In response to these environmental and health concerns, councils in England and Wales are advocating for a ban on single-use vapes by 2024. This proposed ban is driven by issues related to waste management, recycling difficulties, and fire hazards associated with disposable vapes, as well as concerns about their appeal to young people. The UK Vaping Industry Association supports the use of disposable vapes as smoking cessation aids but has raised concerns about the potential rise of black market products if such a ban were to be implemented.

RELATED TECHNOLOGIES

Various devices designed to deliver inhaled nicotine have been developed with the goal of replicating both the ritualistic and behavioral aspects associated with traditional cigarette smoking.

One such innovation involves British American Tobacco, which, through its subsidiary Nicoventures, has adapted a nicotine delivery system using technology originally designed for asthma inhalers. This system, licensed from the UK-based healthcare company Kind Consumer, resulted in the creation of a product named Voke, which received approval from the United Kingdom's Medicines and Healthcare Products Regulatory Agency in September 2014.

In a separate development, Philip Morris International acquired the rights to a nicotine pyruvate technology created by Jed Rose at Duke University in 2011. This technology utilizes a chemical reaction between pyruvic acid and nicotine to produce an inhalable nicotine pyruvate vapor. Additionally, Philip Morris Products S.A. developed a unique e-cigarette model known as the P3L. This device features a cartridge with separate compartments for nicotine and lactic acid. When the device is activated and heated, the nicotine salt, nicotine lactate, is transformed into an aerosol.

The IQOS, a heated tobacco product developed and marketed by Philip Morris International, represents a significant advancement in tobacco consumption technology. Unlike traditional cigarettes, which burn tobacco at high temperatures, the IQOS heats tobacco at a considerably lower temperature, reaching up to 350°C. The product was first introduced to the market in

Japan in November 2014. By December 2016, the United Tobacco Vapor Group (UTVG) announced that it had secured a patent for its innovative vaporizing component system. Notably, UTVG's IQOS does not use a wick or sponge, and its design features only five components, compared to the twenty found in conventional e-cigarettes.

Pax Labs has also contributed to the evolution of nicotine delivery systems with its line of vaporizers designed to heat tobacco leaves and produce vaporized nicotine. In June 2015, Pax Labs launched Juul, an e-cigarette that delivers nicotine at a significantly higher concentration than most other e-cigarettes, matching the nicotine delivery of a traditional cigarette puff. Juul was spun off from Pax Labs in June 2017 to operate as an independent company under the name Juul Labs. Additionally, the eTron 3T, introduced by Vapor Tobacco Manufacturing in December 2014, employs a patented aqueous system that extracts tobacco into water, creating an e-liquid composed of organic tobacco, organic glycerin, and water.

Japan Tobacco introduced the Ploom in December 2013, followed by the launch of Ploom TECH in January 2016. Ploom TECH produces vapor by heating a liquid that passes through a capsule filled with granulated tobacco leaves. British American Tobacco (BAT) also entered the market with its own heat-not-burn product, glo, which was released in Japan and Switzerland in 2016. Unlike traditional smoking methods, glo uses tobacco sticks instead of nicotine liquid and avoids directly heating or burning the tobacco.

The concept of heated tobacco products has been around since 1988, but it only gained commercial traction in recent years. BLOW began offering e-hookahs, an electronic version of the traditional hookah, in 2014. Each e-hookah hose features a heating element and liquid that generates vapor. Gopal Bhatnagar, based in Toronto, Canada, invented a 3D-printed adapter that transforms a traditional hookah into an e-hookah, replacing the ceramic bowl used for shisha tobacco with a mechanism for inserting e-cigarettes. Additionally, KanaVape offers an e-cigarette that contains cannabidiol (CBD) without THC, while companies like Canada's Eagle Energy Vapor are marketing caffeine-based e-cigarettes as an alternative to nicotine products.

CHAPTER FOUR

HOW TO VAPE

Vaping has become a popular alternative to smoking traditional cigarettes. For newcomers, the process of vaping might seem daunting, but understanding the basics can make it a smooth experience. This article provides a step-by-step guide on how to vape, including the essential equipment, techniques, and safety tips.

1. Understanding the Basics

Vaping involves inhaling vapor produced by an electronic device called a vaporizer or e-cigarette. These devices heat a liquid, commonly known as e-liquid or vape juice, which contains nicotine, flavorings, and other ingredients. The heated liquid turns into vapor, which the user then inhales.

2. Choosing Your Equipment

Types of Vaping Devices:

•Cigalikes: These are compact devices resembling traditional cigarettes. They are ideal for beginners due to their simplicity and ease of use.

•Vape Pens: Slightly larger than cigalikes, vape pens offer a longer battery life and more customization options.

•Box Mods: These are advanced devices that offer greater power and customization. They are suitable for experienced vapers.

E-Liquid:

•Nicotine Levels: E-liquids come in various nicotine strengths, ranging from nicotine-free to high concentrations. Choose a nicotine level that suits your preferences.

•Flavors: E-liquids are available in a wide range of flavors, including fruits, desserts, and menthol. Experiment to find your favorite.

3. <u>Assembling and Preparing Your Device</u>

•Charging the Battery: Ensure that your device's battery is fully charged before use. Most devices come with a USB charger that connects to a power source.

•Filling the Tank: For devices with a refillable tank, carefully fill it with e-liquid. Avoid overfilling to prevent leaks. If using a disposable cartridge, simply attach it to the device.

•Priming the Coil: If your device uses replaceable coils, it's essential to prime them before use. Add a few drops of e-liquid directly to the coil to prevent dry hits and extend its lifespan.

4. <u>Vaping Techniques</u>

•Turn On the Device: Most devices have a power button that needs to be pressed several times to activate. Refer to your device's manual for specific instructions.

•Adjust Settings (if applicable): If using a device with adjustable settings, such as wattage or temperature, set them according to your preference. Start with lower settings and gradually increase them.

•Inhaling: Place the mouthpiece between your lips and gently inhale the vapor into your mouth. Avoid taking deep breaths immediately. Instead, allow the vapor to mix with the air in your mouth before inhaling it into your lungs if desired.

•Exhaling: Exhale the vapor slowly. The vapor produced may be dense or light, depending on your device and settings.

5. <u>Maintenance and Safety</u>

•Cleaning: Regularly clean your device to ensure optimal performance. This includes wiping the tank, mouthpiece, and any other removable parts.

•Battery Safety: Handle batteries with care and avoid overcharging them. Store them in a cool, dry place and dispose of them properly.

•E-Liquid Storage: Store e-liquids away from direct sunlight and extreme temperatures. Keep them out of reach of children and pets.

•Replacement Parts: Replace coils and other parts as needed to maintain the device's functionality and flavor quality.

6. <u>Understanding the Regulations</u>

Familiarize yourself with local regulations regarding vaping. Some regions have specific laws governing the use, sale, and advertisement of e-cigarettes and related products. Vaping can be a satisfying and less harmful alternative to smoking when done correctly. By understanding your equipment, practicing proper vaping techniques, and adhering to safety guidelines, you can enhance your vaping experience. Always stay informed about the latest developments in vaping technology and regulations to ensure a safe and enjoyable experience.

119

CONCLUSION

In conclusion, vaping marks a significant shift in the landscape of nicotine consumption, representing a modern and innovative alternative to traditional smoking. With its roots in advanced technology and a diverse array of flavors and devices, vaping caters to a wide range of preferences and needs, from those seeking a less harmful alternative to cigarette smoking to enthusiasts exploring new sensory experiences.

As you delve into the world of vaping, you'll encounter an ever-evolving industry that continues to push the boundaries of what's possible. The array of vaping devices, from simple e-cigarettes to sophisticated mods, offers a customizable experience that allows users to tailor their nicotine intake and flavor profiles to their liking. Understanding the nuances of these devices, the science behind e-liquids, and the proper techniques for use will empower you to make well-informed choices and enhance your vaping journey.

The rise of vaping has not been without its controversies and debates, particularly concerning health implications and regulatory challenges. As the industry grows, staying abreast of the latest research and regulations is crucial for making safe and responsible choices. Vaping, while offering potential benefits over traditional smoking, requires careful consideration and awareness of its effects and legal status.

Ultimately, vaping represents more than just a trend; it embodies a transformative shift in how we approach nicotine consumption. It offers a new horizon for those looking to move away from traditional cigarettes or simply explore a different facet of modern lifestyle choices. By embracing this evolution with curiosity and knowledge, you can navigate the complexities of vaping with confidence, ensuring that your experience is both enjoyable and informed.

As you embark on this journey, remember that vaping is a personal choice influenced by individual preferences and health considerations. With a growing array of products and a dynamic industry landscape, vaping invites you to explore and experiment within a framework of safety and awareness. As the future of vaping continues to unfold, it promises to offer new opportunities for enjoyment and discovery, reflecting the ongoing evolution of nicotine consumption in the 21st century.